Therapeutic Uses of
VEGETABLE JUICES

Titles of Related Interest

Therapeutic Uses of
VEGETABLE JUICES

Dr. Hugo Brandenberger

Keats Publishing, Inc. New Canaan, Connecticut

Therapeutic Uses of Vegetable Juices is not intended as medical advice. Its intent is solely informational and educational. Please consult a health professional should the need for one be indicated.

ISBN: 0-87983-578-8

Printed in the United States of America
Published by Keats Publishing, Inc.
27 Pine Street (Box 876)
New Canaan, Connecticut 06840-0876

Table of Contents

Vegetables and Juices

All the nourishment we take in from our food derives from plants and from the sun, which powers the growth of those plants. Meat and other animal foods are merely an elaboration of plant energy; we eat the substance of animals that produced that substance by eating plants.

When we eat vegetables directly, we are taking in that plant-sun energy in its basic form, and also benefiting from the minerals that the plant has extracted from the earth, several important vitamins, and the fibrous structure necessary to the functioning of the digestive system. There are those who claim that a completely vegetarian diet is the best for humans, others who maintain that animal protein is needed; but most nutrition experts today agree that a very substantial proportion of our diet should be vegetables, preferably raw or very little cooked, as high heat destroys many important nutrients.

Hippocrates, regarded as the first of all physicians, advised, "Let your food be your medicine and your medicine your food," and indeed foods, especially vegetable foods, were among the earliest of remedies for disease. As food and as medicine, garlic, onions and celery root have been valued since before recorded history, and the knowledge of their medical value is still being extended.

When vegetables are juiced, almost all their nutrient content is transferred to the juice, which thereby becomes an extra-potent concentration of nutrients, a therapeutic substance rather than a merely nutritional one. It should be noted that the maximum benefits of vegetable juices are realized only when they are derived from organically grown vegetables. Such vegetables are free from sometimes harmful pesticide residues and contain a natural balance of the complete range of soil nutrients, which are not present in commercially fertilized vegetables.

Many practitioners of natural medicine have used juice therapy to heal or relieve serious conditions, from digestive problems to life-threatening diseases such as cancer, and scientific researchers have explored and verified many of the therapeutic

7

properties possessed by vegetable juices. This booklet will examine some of these juices and how they are employed to maintain or restore health, concluding with an examination of a remarkable combination of juices which has shown great effectiveness in the treatment of many forms of cancer.

Lactofermentation

Most of us are familiar with a wide variety of juices, mainly fruit juices. There is fresh-squeezed orange juice from the kitchen, canned tomato juice, frozen apple juice concentrate, grapefruit juice in a carton, mixtures of cranberry and other juices in half-gallon bottles. And then there are "juice drinks," mainly water, flavored with substances that may or may not be natural fruit juices. Vegetable juices are much less widely known, and the chances are that your exposure, if any, has been to carrot juice served at a health-food bar. Home juicers are becoming popular, and many people are discovering the taste and benefit of fresh, home-prepared juices.

However, good juicers are substantial investments, and the process is time-consuming and at least somewhat troublesome; and in general fresh juices do not keep well, so that you can't make up several days' supply at one time. Convenience in obtaining vegetable juices of high quality and having them on hand ready to drink when you want them requires a method of preserving the juices. The standard commercial method is to sterilize the juice by heating it to 248° Fahrenheit. This kills the bacteria that would make the juice spoil—but at the same time severely impairs the vitamins and other active agents contained in the fresh vegetables. This is one reason you do not see cans or bottles of celery root or carrot juice on your supermarket shelves: the process that would preserve them would make them much less worth drinking.

There is a natural preservative method which does not require heating to this extreme extent: lactofermentation, fermentation by the agency of lactic acid bacteria. This is what preserves and indeed enhances the nutrient values in milk by turning it to yogurt, or cabbage by turning it into sauerkraut.

This brings up an obvious drawback. Yogurt and sauerkraut,

however wholesome and in their own way appetizing, are definitely sour, and this is the result of lactofermentation. Vegetable juices subjected to the full process of lactofermentation will have a taste more or less reminiscent of sauerkraut, and it appears to be a taste not many are willing to learn to like.

Whey, the milk "serum"—perhaps familiar to you as the watery substance that exudes from the solid portions of yogurt—contains lactic acid, and it has been found that adding whey to vegetable juices gives the preservative effect of lactofermentation without altering the natural taste of the original vegetables. Juices preserved in this manner can be shipped and stored for extended periods of time without loss of flavor or nutritional value, and without resort to sterilization or chemicals.

The whey contains neither fat nor casein, and so adds no significant amount of calories to the juice. It does add significant nutritional value, though. Dr. H. Anemüller, a well-known diet specialist, writes that whey "contains a little high-grade protein, and is above all rich in lactose, B group vitamins and minerals. Especially important is the wealth of potassium contained in whey, which activates an extrusion of sodium and acid metabolic products." Dr. Anemüller notes that the taste of whey is highly compatible with those of vegetable juices. Whey's content of lactobacilli is also considered to give it a preventative effect against the degeneration of the intestinal flora, a major cause of digestive problems.

The different juices treated in this work are most readily available as lactofermented preparations, and we will be discussing their benefits and properties primarily in that form. In his encyclopedic work on natural health, *The Nature Doctor,* Dr. Alfred Vogel observes: "Lactic acid is a fine healing factor for the intestines. Juices that are fermented with lactic acid are more easily tolerated than freshly pressed ones, and it is possible to take at least one-third more of the lactic-fermented juices than of those prepared from fresh produce at home."

Sauerkraut Juice

As we mentioned earlier, one of the most familiar examples of lactofermentation is sauerkraut, fermented cabbage. The other juices to be discussed in this work have been subjected to a mild form of lactofermentation through the use of whey, but sauerkraut receives the full treatment, and derives many of its health benefits from that. Sauerkraut juice has enjoyed for centuries the reputation of being a powerful natural medicine, in great part because of its high lactic acid content.

Lactic Acid

Lactic acid is a powerful systemic disinfectant, and is useful in cases of hydrochloric acid deficiency, which can affect both children and the elderly more often than is usually realized. It acts by improving the protein complex in the stomach and by speeding up the transformation of ferrous compounds into organic iron.

Carbohydrates, absorbed through the intestine, are transformed into lactic acid before being stored in the liver as glycogen. Any impairment of liver function interferes with this vital process, and the lactic acid content of sauerkraut juice is often useful to those experiencing liver trouble and other metabolic disturbances. Lactic acid is sometimes given intravenously to liver patients as a protective measure.

Traditional folk medical lore in Europe has long held that eating sauerkraut promotes growth in children, and a high lactic acid content has been observed in the blood of rapidly growing children. At the other end of life, the effects of lactofermented foods on old people were noted by scientists as long ago as 1739, when the longevity and good health of the Wallachians in Romania was ascribed to the prevalence of sauerkraut and soured milk products in their diet.

Other Properties

Sauerkraut juice is well known as a laxative. This is considered to be the result both of its high acetylcholine content and of the fact that sauerkraut contains about 1.5 percent natural lactic acid that normalizes intestinal flora and destroys pathogenic bacteria in the intestinal tract, stimulating peristaltic action. Sauerkraut juice is also therefore useful in dealing with the side effects of constipation, such as headaches. It has been used successfully to rid patients of worms, particularly infestations of nematodes in children, but this may well be associated with its laxative properties, as no specific vermicidal substance for intestinal worms has been discovered in sauerkraut or its juice.

Sauerkraut is high in magnesium, potassium and calcium, and these minerals are believed to account for its diuretic properties.

Most of the sugar-building carbohydrates present in the cabbage from which sauerkraut is made are destroyed during the fermentation process, so that the calorie content is low, making it suitable for diabetic diets.

Hemorrhoids have been benefited by sauerkraut juice, and vomiting during pregnancy can often be soothed with a few swallows.

Recent medical research has demonstrated anticancer properties in vegetables of the brassica family, which includes cabbage, from which sauerkraut is made, though no research has been done in this area specifically involving sauerkraut.

Scurvy is no longer the scourge that it was centuries ago, when it killed thousands of sailors and other travelers cut off from fresh vegetables, but modern processed diets often produce a "hidden" scurvy, manifested by spongy or bleeding gums, joint swelling and fatigue. The antiscorbutic properties of citrus fruits are well known, but cabbage and sauerkraut are highly effective scurvy fighters. The 18th-century explorer Captain Cook used fermented cabbage to keep his sailors alive for years at sea; and Genghis Khan is said to have kept his Mongol horsemen healthy enough to conquer much of Europe by filling their saddlebags with sauerkraut.

The antiscorbutic factor in cabbage and sauerkraut is now known to be vitamin C, new benefits of which are constantly being discovered. It is, for one thing, a major antioxidant and consequently an important defense against many varieties of degenerative diseases and the effects of the aging process.

Beetroot Juice

The dark red juice of the beet, powerful enough to color a quart of water with a few drops, has been associated with blood since antiquity. The early physicians Galen and Dioscurides considered beet juice medically important for its blood-building and healing properties, and modern research has confirmed their existence with analyses showing the presence of an abundance of potassium, sulfur, iodine, iron and copper. While the quantity of iron is not great, the concurrent presence of trace elements make it unusually bioavailable and therefore, as the ancient healers believed, beneficial to red blood cell growth. Beets also contain the B vitamin complex, including niacin and choline, vitamins A, C and P, useful quantities of amino acids, and betaine, which, according to Dr. Alfred Vogel, "stimulates the function of the liver cells and protects the liver and bile ducts in cases of disturbance." In his classic work, *The Nature Doctor,* Dr. Vogel particularly recommends beet juice "in the first two years of life, during puberty, in pregnancy, when breast-feeding and during the menopause."

In *The Juicing Book,* health researcher Stephen Blauer lists these conditions that are responsive to beet juice therapy: anemia, bladder disorders, cancer, circulatory problems, fatigue, heart disease, both hypertension and hypotension, liver and kidney disorders, menstrual problems and skin conditions.

Cancer-Fighting Properties

In the 1950s the Hungarian physician and scientist Dr. Alexander Ferenczi pioneered research in the anticancer properties of beet juice. Dr. Ferenczi observed that a colleague had used beet juice successfully in the treatment of leukemia patients, and, knowing that substances effective against leukemia are often effective against tumors as well, performed laboratory experiments with beet juice on rats injected with tumorigenic substances. These were successful enough so that a clinical trial on human patients was justified.

The first group consisted of 22 patients, all with advanced, inoperable cancers. Each patient received 3 deciliters (about 10 ounces) of beet juice a day, and after 3 to 4 months, 21 patients showed marked improvement, manifested in diminution of the tumor, weight increase of up to 24 pounds, and normalization of the rate of blood sedimentation.

Dr. Ferenczi theorized that an active ingredient in the beet juice replaced a necessary substance in the patients' tissues that had been depleted by cancerous changes in the cells. He observed that it was a natural, harmless remedy of apparent efficacy and possessed of no side effects, and of course inexpensive and available in unlimited quantities.

The lactic acid content of lactofermented forms of beet juice also appears important in promoting good health and preventing cancer formation.

An article by Dr. P. D. Seeger of Berlin in the journal *Vitalstoffe* (Issue 5/1966) reported on Dr. Ferenczi's work and on that of Dr. S. Schmidt, who "achieved good results" with 50 cancer patients and 15 leukemia patients; it also noted other researchers' discovery of a growth-retarding and growth-inhibiting effect of beet juice on cancer cells. Of his own work, in collaboration with Dr. Schacht, Dr. Seeger wrote that

> using combined treatment of cytostatics [substances that hinder cell growth] and breathing activators (hydrogen acceptors and organic acids) on cancerous mice in 1962, [the experimenters] achieved an experimental mouse life span 18-20 times longer.
>
> Due to the action of its protective coloring matter (cyanidin, betanidin), its vitamins, minerals, trace elements and ferments, beet juice offers us an ideal cancer preventive and/or cure, which serves as the best substituting mechanism for the inactive respiratory chain of the cancer cells and for the disturbed metabolic functioning. During the months when fresh beet juice is not available, lactofermented beet juice should have top priority, since it contains all the substances (except peroxidase) found in fresh juice, in addition to lactic acid. This combination has shown superior results in our experiments.
>
> Taking our findings into consideration, it appears that a combined dosage of beet juice (fresh or lactofermented) with respiration activators and cytostatics offers the best chance for successful treatment of cancer at this time.
>
> Respiration of the cancerous cells through fresh beet juice is 1000-1250 percent reactivated, i.e., normalized. The workings of beet juice correspond exactly with those indicated by nature for the body's own defense against cancer.

Beet juice's content of vitamin B12 and folic acid are thought to account for its observed efficacy in cases of leukemia, as they contribute to the regeneration of red blood corpuscles. These nutrients may well also account for the effectiveness of beet juice in cases of X-ray or radiation damage, reported to the Eighth International Congress for Preventive Medicine.

Carrot Juice

Like the beet, the carrot has been respected for its medicinal as well as its food value for thousands of years. The Greeks called it philon, because of its supposed value as an aphrodisiac; but if it has any value in that area, it is probably because of its beneficial effects on all aspects of health. In *The Juicing Book*, Stephen Blauer refers to it as "the king of vegetable juices," and it is certainly one of the most powerful.

Carrot Power

Dr. William Lee's *Book of Raw Fruit and Vegetable Juices and Drinks* credits carrot juice with providing energy, serving as a source of important minerals, promoting normal elimination, diuretic properties, building healthy tissue, skin and teeth, stimulating appetite, preventing mucous membrane and eye infections, and aiding in the treatment of ulcers.

Carrot juice has a strong effect on the digestive system through the essential oils it contains; its content of alkaline minerals, especially calcium and magnesium, is also important. These benefit the mucous membranes and stimulate circulation of the blood in the tissues of the intestines and stomach. It works against both diarrhea and constipation, exercising a regularizing effect, and helps eliminate intestinal worms.

Certain skin complaints are associated with digestive problems—e.g., eczema and acne—and can be relieved with the use of carrot juice, as can some forms of headache. Many use it as an internally taken "beauty treatment," and are happy with the results; it both benefits skin health and promotes loss of excessive weight. Provitamin A activates melanin, which is responsible for pigmentation in the skin, and can promote the development of a pleasing tan with less exposure to the sun.

Drinking excessive amounts of carrot juice has been known

to darken or yellow the skin somewhat, but reducing the intake of carrot juice solves the problem quickly.

Regular use of carrot juice is reported to aid liver function and promote the excretion of bile and excess fat, thus reducing blood cholesterol levels.

It is regarded almost universally as a superior all-round tonic, and is recommended for use during convalescence after surgery or serious illness, colds and fever. Arthritis, cancer, diabetes, hay fever and ulcers are among the conditions reported as responsive to carrot juice in Blauer's *Juicing Book.* In *The Nature Doctor,* Dr. Vogel recommends carrot juice as a remedy for overcoming calcium deficiency in children, and as part of regimens for impaired liver function, heart disease and obesity caused by endocrine gland malfunctioning.

The most popular belief about carrots and carrot juice is that they promote good eyesight, and, unlike many things "everybody knows," this belief is correct. The high carotene (provitamin A) content of both the vegetable and the juice both benefits the mucous membranes of the eye, as mentioned above, and stimulates the production of rhodopsin, a substance required for adequate night vision. Dr. Vogel further observes: "It is a proven fact that a carrot juice diet has a favorable effect on the eyes on account of the provitamin A carrots contain. Anything that stimulates the circulation and the supply of blood to the eyes helps improve their efficiency, and this is where carrot juice is most beneficial."

The "Nature Doctor's" Comments

Elsewhere in his authoritative book, Dr. Vogel has much to say about the benefits of carrots, carrot juice and carotene:

> Carrots are so rich in important minerals and vitamins that they can rightly be called a remedial food. You should eat them every day in one form or another, especially during the low-vitamin winter months and early spring.

He notes the high content of potassium, calcium, iron and copper, and pays special attention to the phosphorus content of carrots:

> . . . we all appreciate the importance of phosphorus for our brain, particularly our memory. Carrots are also good for the

glands because of their content of iodine. Furthermore, they are a source of magnesium and cobalt, as well as carotene (provitamin A) at the rate of 70 mg per kilogram of carrots.

Carotene is extremely important in our effort to keep the cellular system healthy and the digestive organs functioning efficiently. It promotes healthy growth and the development of strong, resistant teeth. In fact, vitamin A, that is, carotene, together with calcium and vitamin D, contributes considerably to good teeth.

Did you know, too, that carotene, if taken plentifully, is able to prevent the formation of kidney stones? This has been proven by careful observations. And another thing, a lack of carotene is one of the factors that contributes to a greater susceptibility to infections, especially coughs and sneezes.

Taking plenty of carotene helps to achieve a faster and more complete recovery in cases of pneumonia, various heart troubles, eczema and psoriasis. Women should also take greater amounts of it during pregnancy. It is generally known that it is good for the eyes, helping to improve the eyesight and, if taken in sufficient quantities, it can be the means of overcoming night-blindness—a tremendous benefit to pilots and night-drivers. [Author's note: We should also note that the very large group of people who watch television a great deal or work long hours at computer screens will be enormously helped by carotene.] Carotene has another welcome benefit in that it reduces the tendency to form cataracts. In addition, experiments and observations have shown that carotene improves the function of the sex glands because it exerts a certain influence on the production of sex hormones; thus it can be of assistance in overcoming sexual weakness and impotence. This effect may be attributable to the high vitamin E content in carrots . . . Finally, just let me mention some other vitamins in carrots: . . . vitamins B1, B2 and B6, as well as the important vitamin K, and . . . vitamin C, the valuable nerve food.

Celery Root Juice

A close relative of parsley, celery root was used centuries ago as a diuretic and laxative, as a wound healer and a natural tranquilizer, and to expel gallstones. Its strong concentration of plant hormones and essential oils, which give it its characteristic "fresh" odor, together with its high concentration of alkaline minerals such as sodium, appear to regulate and calm the central nervous system. These attributes have earned it the name of "European ginseng," after the famous tonic and therapeutic Asian herb.

Its calming property accounts for celery root juice's popularity as a tonic and relaxant. A glass of celery root juice, with a teaspoon of honey, is said to help control a dieter's appetite if sipped slowly before eating. The juice is also known as an excellent blood cleanser, and promotes the discharge of toxins from the system. While it is used for its stimulating effect on the sexual system, it acts to normalize function in this regard, and may compensate for a weakened sex drive without making an active one overactive. Asthma, bronchitis, constipation, insomnia and weight loss are among other conditions reported by Blauer in *The Juicing Book* to be responsive to celery root juice.

Relief for Rheumatism and Arthritis

Its alkalinity and diuretic properties have given celery root juice a reputation for effectiveness in dealing with rheumatism and arthritis. Dr. Alfred Vogel writes: "Celery root juice is distinctly alkaline and eliminative. It is therefore recommended for all disturbances caused by the accumulation of wastes and toxins, for example rheumatic and arthritic ailments. Celery juice regulates the water balance and puts new life in elderly people." Dr. P. D. Seeger, quoted earlier on the therapeutic effects of beet juice, states that celery root juice "has a diuretic effect and can be recommended for circulatory disturbances and heart disease, for rheumatism and calculosis." The alkaline content helps to prevent buildup of excessive acid in the blood, a great contributor to these conditions.

Dr. Ernst Schneider, in his book *Use the Healing Force of Our Nutrition*, states that celery root juice's

> content of essential oils is responsible for the therapeutic effect on the kidney vasculars. They are dilated and the water secretion is higher. With this higher secretion toxic metabolic products can be discharged: hence the good effect on gout, rheumatism, proneness to calculus formation and acidity in lesions.

Walther Schoenenberger in *Natural Juices* proclaims its benefits firmly:

> Celery root juice is the strongest stimulus for the whole kidney function. It is a natural help for better secretion of metabolic bulk and brings about a significant discharge of the coherent manifestations such as gout and arthritis; celery root juice is also indicated for calculosis and edema or kidney hypofunction.

Potato Juice

Like the tomato, the potato was brought from the New World to a fairly suspicious Old World that harbored for a long time the idea that the new vegetable was poisonous. Though potatoes are related to the nightshade family, and can develop dangerous toxins under certain conditions, they are now almost the most necessary and widespread of all vegetable foods, rivaled only by some grains.

The potato's mixture of carbohydrates, protein, lipids, vitamins and minerals is what gives it its unique nutritional value, making it nearly a complete meal in itself. The potato is also outstandingly effective therapeutically, grated or mashed potatoes being used as poultices to deal with inflammations, infections, slowly healing wounds, bruises, muscular inflammation and arthritis.

It is therefore not surprising that potato juice is also useful in the treatment of many ailments. Like celery root juice, it is effective against arthritis, and indeed Dr. Alfred Vogel calls it "the most important remedy" for this disease, noting that it is "not only its alkaline constituents which contribute to curing arthritis but possibly other, as yet unknown, factors."

Relief for Ulcers and Other Gastric Problems

Wars sometimes bring unexpected benefits and advances, particularly in medicine, when new ways of saving lives under crisis conditions are desperately sought, and drastic changes in living patterns show unexpected results. The reduction in meats and fats in the diets of many populations during the Second World War, for instance, brought about a decrease in

degenerative diseases and heart conditions, providing important new information on the role of diet in disease. And some
groups of German soldiers in World War I, near starvation
and forced to live on raw potatoes they dug from the shell-
ploughed fields, found that any gastric disorders, such as ulcers, they suffered from were relieved or cured. As ulcers were
associated strongly with stress, their healing under conditions
of ultimate stress was unexpected and highly interesting.

After the war, Dr. J. F. Magerl looked into this curious piece
of battlefield medical lore, and began treating gastric patients
with raw potato juice. Nearly 90 percent of the patients re-
sponded favorably by the second day of the treatment, and
most showed no symptoms after 10 days.

One theoretical explanation for this remarkable effect is that
the solanin in potatoes inhibits the over-secretion of gastric
fluids, which is the cause of ulcers and most gastric distress,
and that their starch, minerals and lipids soothe and seal the
stomach's mucous membrane with a protective buffering action. Potatoes' high vitamin C content also helps inhibit infec-
tion during treatment.

For heartburn, caused by the reflux of digestive fluids into
the throat area, the first remedy Dr. Alfred Vogel suggests is
potato juice, which he recommends as effective in all gastric
conditions. Like Dr. Magerl, he has learned that "taken regu-
larly it has a marvelous healing effect" on stomach ulcers,
which "usually disappear within 3-6 weeks."

Some Healed Patients

A British journalist, Jack Temple, became curious after en-
countering stories of the ulcer-healing properties of potato juice,
and traveled to Switzerland to interview former ulcer sufferers.
He garnered many stories, of which we will here give four:

Robert Senn, mayor of the town of Kreuzlingen, lived a high-
pressure business life, which by the time he reached 55 had
provided him with the businessman's standard ailment, a full-
blown set of stomach ulcers. A month after a friend persuaded
him to start a potato juice treatment, the ulcers were gone, and
he had at the time of the interview been free of them for 10

years, during each day of which he had had his daily dose of the lactofermented potato juice.

Richard Boder, in his late 20s, collapsed with unbearable pain brought about by extreme stomach acidity; his episodes of pain coincided with periods of intense anger. After four days on potato juice, the pain was relieved, and had not returned during five years of a daily glassful of juice.

Relief came even faster, within two days, to Dr. H. Dorstewitz, who treated his acute gastritis with potato juice; the condition had not recurred during the time preceding the interview, about a year.

Lisa Straub, 76 when interviewed, did not look as if she had suffered from an incapacitating duodenal ulcer 13 years before. She had read something about the curative powers of potato juice, and got some potatoes and juiced them. The results were not good, and Mrs. Straub believed that it was because the potatoes were not organically produced. She then tried the juice in its organically grown, lactofermented, bottled form, and enjoyed much more success. About four ounces a day, sipped early in the morning, relieved the pains completely in short order.

A Cancer-Fighting Juice Combination

It is axiomatic that almost no nutrient or food is most effective in isolation—that "cooperation" between them produces the best results, with one reinforcing another's benefits. Many of the juices discussed earlier are often used together, e.g., potato and carrot, a combination Dr. Alfred Vogel recommends for the treatment of stomach ulcers.

One of the most remarkable of juice combinations, which is reported to have helped many thousands of people, is Rudolf Breuss's anticancer mixture. Its composition is simple:

Beetroot	55%
Celery root	20
Carrot	20
Potato	3
Radish	2

As we have seen, each of these juices has important medicinal effects, from beetroot juice's specific action on cancer to potato juice's promotion of gastric health. Together, in the fasting regimen developed by Breuss, in which only the juices and some herbs are taken, they appear to exert a powerful therapeutic effect on cancer, as attested to by the more than 24,000 patients who wrote to him detailing the relief from their diseases that the treatment had brought them.

An Austrian, Rudolf Breuss died in 1989 at the age of 93. In the early 1950s he developed through extensive research a natural, drugless six-week treatment for cancer, based on the concept that the cancerous tumor, being composed of protein, needs a supply of protein in order to survive and grow.

The patient is given approximately half a pint of the juices a day in small doses. The beetroot juice is particularly valuable in enhancing cell respiration; the celery root juice promotes body cleansing, the potato and carrot juices benefit the stomach and the radish juice the gallbladder. The juice combination is taken with teas made from many herbs, including nettles, St. John's wort, marigold, artemisia and monarda. The herbs combine with the juices to keep the body's organs working properly in the absence of the usual food supply. The body draws on its protein reserves during this time, successfully competing with and "starving out" the malignant tumor.

The treatment takes 42 days, and at its conclusion the vast majority of those who followed it faithfully are reported to be cured. Rudolf Breuss reported a 96% success rate for the many thousands of patients he treated during his nearly 30 years of practice. Many practitioners and clinics, particularly in Switzerland and Germany, have used the Breuss regimen with excellent results.

Freed from Cancer

Sonja Haubenschmid's recommendation for use of the Breuss juices carry an extra weight of conviction. Mrs. Haubenschmid, who with her microbiologist husband runs a natural therapy clinic in the Swiss town of Amriswil, undertook the treatment herself for a breast cancer from which she had suffered for two years, and was free of it after the prescribed six weeks. During the treatment, her husband photographed the changes occurring in her blood cells, documenting the effects of the juice therapy on them as the cancerous cells disappeared.

Equally remarkable are the five X-ray plates showing the reversal of lung cancer in one of Rudolf Breuss's patients, Mr. Artho. The first plate shows his left lung engulfed by the cancerous growth; at this time he was given four months to live. The succeeding plates chronicle the reappearance of healthy lung tissue and the dwindling of the cancer. When interviewed two years after the treatment he was healthy, active and cancer-free.

Other patients have reported excellent health for up to 30 years after the Breuss treatment for cancers of the breast, brain, colon and lung.

For many of the years he practiced, Rudolf Breuss farmed his own herbs and vegetables on a plot of about 17 acres, and patients who came to consult him were given fresh herbs or freshly pressed vegetable juices especially prescribed for their individual problems. The herbs and vegetables were grown organically, with no chemical fertilizers or pesticides. Breuss devised his own fertilizer from nettles soaked in water, which he believed substantially enriched the medicinal value of his crop. When Rudolf Breuss found it impossible to supply the vegetable juices in the quantity required by the growing number of patients using his regimen, he arranged for their production and bottling in lactofermented form by Biotta, the firm I have the honor to head, insisting that the vegetables from which the juices were derived should continue to be grown according to the organic principles he himself followed.

Conclusion

The tremendous curative power of nature is nowhere better demonstrated than in the vegetable foods the earth provides, which furnish our food and our most effective medicine as well. This power is concentrated in fresh or ferment-preserved juices, which can be used to maintain or regain health, even when the most serious diseases are involved. This book is provided with the intention of introducing its readers to the health-promoting properties of juices and inducing them to see how they can best use these juices in their own lives.

Quick Reference Chart for Healing Juices and Ailments They Affect

This listing shows the juices which have been reported from different sources to have shown effectiveness in cases of the conditions mentioned; it is not intended as recommendation for any self-treatment but as a guide to investigation.

Anemia	beet
Arthritis	celery root, potato
Cancer, leukemia	beet, Breuss formula
Constipation	sauerkraut, carrot, celery root
Diarrhea	carrot
Eczema, skin problems	sauerkraut, carrot
Goiter	sauerkraut
Headache	sauerkraut, carrot
Heartburn	potato
Hemorrhoids	sauerkraut
Infection	sauerkraut, potato
Kidney problems	carrot, celery root
Liver problems	sauerkraut, beet, carrot, radish
Metabolic disturbances	sauerkraut
Nervousness	celery root
Night blindness	carrot
Radiation damage	beet
Scurvy	sauerkraut
Sexual weakness or imbalance	carrot, celery root
Toxemia	celery root
Ulcers	potato
Worms	sauerkraut

Bibliography

Stephen Blauer, *The Juicing Book*. Garden City Park, N.Y.: Avery Publishing Group, 1989.

William H. Lee, R.Ph., Ph.D., *The Book of Raw Fruit and Vegetable Juices and Drinks*. New Canaan, Conn.: Keats Publishing, 1982.

Ernst Schneider, Dr.med., *Use the Healing Force of Our Nutrition (Die Heilkraft unserer Nahrung)*. Hamburg: Saatkorn Verlag, 1978.

Walther Schoenenberger, *Natural Juices (Naturreine Pflanzensäfte)*. Stuttgart: Science Dept. Plant Juice Factory W. Schoenenberger, 1960.

Dr.h.c. Alfred Vogel, *The Nature Doctor (Der kleine Doktor)*. New Canaan, Conn.: Keats Publishing, 1991.